Mediterranean Diet Recipes

Simple and Delicious Recipes For Beginners

By Jenna Wilkinson

Sommario

Introduction

The Mediterranean Diet plan comprises a collection of understanding and also practices varying from landscape to table, consisting of plants, harvesting, angling, preservation, handling, prep work, and also usage of food. It is defined by a dietary design that has actually continued to be continuous in time and also locations, being primarily comprised of: olive oil, grains, fresh and also dried out fruits, veggies, a modest quantity of fish, milk items, meat, several flavorings, as well as flavors, completely accompanied by a glass of wine. It is a version of a lasting diet regimen, as it adds to maintain: high quality, food, and also dietary security and also at the same time advertises the administration of ecological as well as territorial sources. Mediterranean diet regimen is a certain diet regimen by getting rid of refined foods as well as high in hydrogenated fats. It's not always concerning reducing weight, however instead a healthy and balanced way of living selection. It has to do with consuming standard components taken in by those that have actually stayed in the Mediterranean container for a very long time. This is a diet plan abundant in fruits, veggies, and also fish. Food preparation with olive oil is an essential active ingredient as well as is a suitable substitute for hydrogenated fats. Researches reveal that individuals that reside in these areas live longer as well as much better lives.

CHAPTER 5: MEAT RECIPES

Pork and Prunes Stew

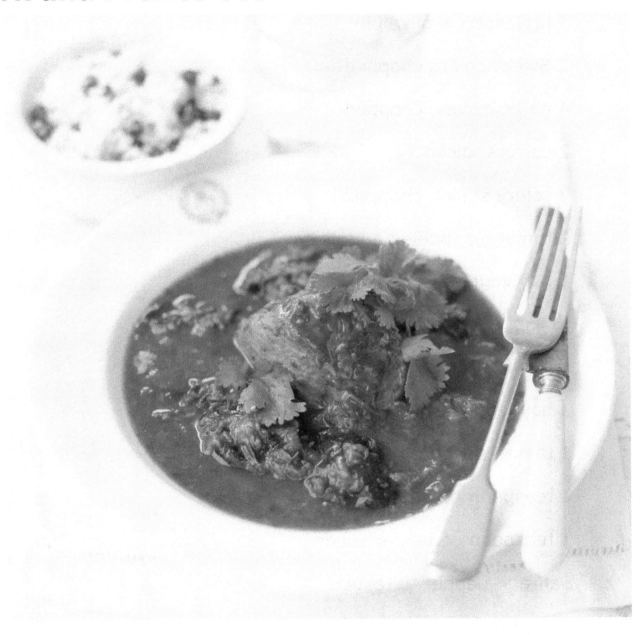

Servings: 8

Preparation time: 1 ¼ Hours

INGREDIENTS

2 pounds pork tenderloin, cubed

2 tablespoons olive oil

1 Sweet onion, chopped

4 garlic cloves, chopped

2 carrots, diced

2 celery stalks, chopped

2 tomatoes, peeled and diced

1 cup vegetable stock

½ cup white wine

1 pound prunes, pitted

1 bay leaf

1 thyme spring

1 teaspoon mustard seeds

1 teaspoon coriander seeds

Salt and pepper to taste

DIRECTIONS

1. Combine all the ingredients in a deep dish baking pan.

2. Add salt and pepper to taste and cook in the preheated oven at 350F for 1 hour, adding more liquid as it cooks if needed.

3. Serve and stew warm and fresh.

NUTRITION: Calories 363, Fat 7.9g, Protein 31.7g, Carbs 41.4g

Pork And Rice Soup

Servings: 4

Preparation time: 7 Hours

INGREDIENTS

- 2 pounds pork stew meat, cubed

- A pinch of salt and black pepper

- 6 cups water

- 1 leek, sliced

- 1 bay leaves

- 1 carrot, sliced

- 3 tablespoons olive oil

- 1 cup white rice

- 2 cups yellow onion, chopped

- ½ cup lemon juice

- 1 tablespoon cilantro, chopped

DIRECTIONS

In your slow cooker, combine the pork with the water and the rest of the ingredients except the cilantro, put the lid on, and cook on Low for 7 hours.

Stir the soup, ladle into bowls, sprinkle the cilantro on top, and serve.

NUTRITION: Calories 300, Fat 15g, Fiber 7.6g, Carbs 17.4g, Protein 22.4g

Sage Pork And Beans Stew

Servings: 4

Preparation time: 4 Hours and 10 minutes

INGREDIENTS

- 2 pounds pork stew meat, cubed
- 2 tablespoons olive oil
- 1 Sweet onion, chopped
- 1 red bell pepper, chopped
- 3 Garlic cloves, minced
- 2 teaspoons sage, dried
- 4 ounces canned white beans, drained
- 1 cup beef stock
- 2 zucchinis, chopped
- 2 tablespoons tomato paste
- 1 tablespoon cilantro, chopped

DIRECTIONS

1. Heat up a pan with the oil over medium-high heat, add the meat, brown for 10 minutes, and transfer to your slow cooker.

2. Add the rest of the ingredients except the cilantro, put the lid on, and cook on High for 4 hours.

3. Divide the stew into bowls, sprinkle the cilantro on top, and serve

NUTRITION: Calories 423, Fat 15.4g, Fiber 9.6g, Carbs 2704g, Protein 43g

Pear Braised Pork

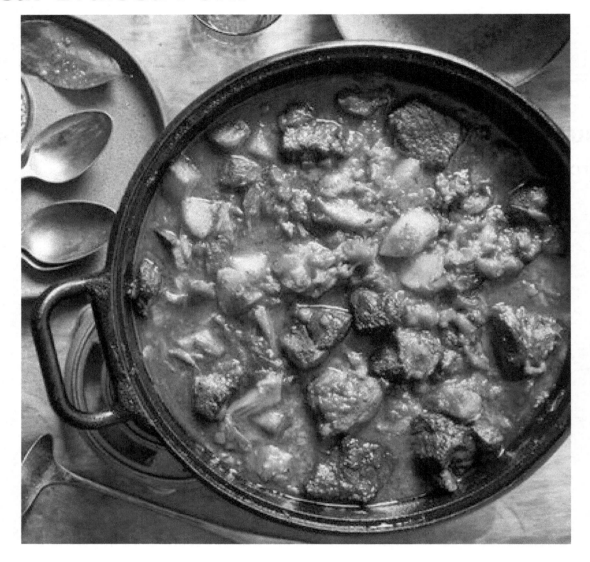

Servings: 10

Preparation time: 2 ¼ hours

INGREDIENTS

- 3 pounds pork shoulder

- 4 Pears, peeled and sliced

- 2 shallots, sliced

- 4 garlic cloves, minced

- 1 bay leaf

- 1 thyme spring

- ½ cup apple cider

- Salt and pepper to taste

DIRECTIONS

1. Season the pork with salt and pepper.

2. Combine the pears, shallots, garlic, bay leaf, thyme, and apple cider in a deep dish baking pan.

3. Place the pork over the pears, then cover the pan with aluminum foil.

4. Cook in the preheated oven at 330F for 2 hours. Serve the pork and the sauce fresh.

NUTRITION: Calories 455, Fat 29.3g, Protein 32.1g, Carbs 14.9g

Tasty Beef Stew

Servings: 4

Preparation time: 30 minutes

INGREDIENTS

2 ½ lbs beef roast, cut into chunks

1 cup beef broth

½ cup balsamic vinegar

1 tbsp honey

½ tsp red pepper flakes

1 tbsp garlic, minced

Pepper

Salt

DIRECTIONS

1. Add all ingredients into the inner pot of the instant pot and stir well.

2. Seal pot with lid and cook on high for 30 minutes.

3. Once done, allow to release pressure naturally. Remove lid.

4. Stir well and serve.

NUTRITION: Calories 562, Fat 18g, Carbs 5.7g, Sugar 4.6g, Protein 87.5g, Cholesterol 253mg

Pork And Sage Couscous

Servings: 4

Preparation time: 7 Hours

INGREDIENTS

- 2 pounds pork loin boneless and sliced
- ¾ cup veggie stock
- 2 tablespoons olive oil
- ½ tablespoon chili powder
- 2 teaspoon sage, dried
- ½ tablespoon garlic powder
- Salt and black pepper to the taste
- 2 cups couscous, cooked

DIRECTIONS

In a slow cooker, combine the pork with the stock and the other ingredients except for the couscous, put the lid on, and cook on low for 7 hours.

Divide the mix between plates, add the couscous on the side, sprinkle the sage on top, and serve.

NUTRITION: Calories 270, Fat 14.5g, Fiber 9g, Carbs 16.3g, Protein 14.3g

Beef And Potatoes With Tahini Sauce

Servings: 1/6 Casserole

Preparation time: 35 minutes

INGREDIENTS

½ large yellow onion

1 lb. ground beef

½ tsp. salt

½ tsp. ground black pepper

6 small red potatoes, washed

3 TB. extra-virgin olive oil

2 cups plain Greek yogurt

¾ cup tahini paste

1½ cups water

¼ cup fresh lemon juice

1 TB. minced garlic

½ cup pine nuts

DIRECTIONS

Preheat the oven to 425°F.

In a food processor fitted with a chopping blade, blend yellow onion for 30 seconds.

Transfer onion to a large bowl. Add beef, 1 teaspoon salt, black pepper, and mix well.

Spread beef mixture evenly in the bottom of a 9-inch casserole dish, and bake for 20 minutes.

Cut red potatoes into 1/4-inch-thick pieces, place in a bowl, and toss with 2 tablespoons extra-virgin olive oil and ½ teaspoon salt.

Spread potatoes on a baking sheet and bake for 20 minutes.

In a large bowl, combine Greek yogurt, tahini paste, water, lemon juice, garlic, and the remaining 1 teaspoon salt.

Remove beef mixture and potatoes from the oven. Using a spatula, transfer potatoes to the casserole dish. Pour yogurt sauce over the top and bake for 15 more minutes.

In a small pan over low heat, heat the remaining 1 tablespoon extra- virgin olive oil. Add pine nuts and toast for 1 or 2 minutes.

Remove casserole dish from the oven, spoon pine nuts over the top and serve warm with brown rice.

NUTRITION Calories 342, Fat 11g, Protein 31g, Carbs 30g, Fiber 6g

Spicy Beef Chili Verde

Servings: 2

Preparation time: 23 minutes

INGREDIENTS

- ½ lb beef stew meat, cut into cubes
- ¼ tsp chili powder
- 1 tbsp olive oil
- 1 cup chicken broth
- 1 Serrano pepper. chopped
- 1 tsp garlic, minced
- 1 small onion, chopped
- ½ cup grape tomatoes, chopped
- ½ cup tomatillos, chopped
- Pepper
- Salt

DIRECTIONS

Add oil into the instant pot and set the pot on sauté mode.

Add garlic and onion and sauté for 3 minutes. Add remaining ingredients and stir well.

Seal pot with lid and cook on high for 20 minutes. Once done, allow to release pressure naturally. Remove lid.

Stir well and serve.

NUTRITION: Calories 317, Fat 15g, Carbs 6.4g, Sugar 2.6g, Protein 37g, Cholesterol 100mg

Coriander Pork And Chickpeas Stew

Servings: 4

Preparation Time: 8 Hours

INGREDIENTS

- ½ cup beef stock

- 1 tablespoon ginger, grated

- 1 teaspoon coriander. ground

- z teaspoons cumin, ground

- Salt and black pepper to the taste

- 2 and ½ pounds pork stew meat, cubed

- 28 ounces canned tomatoes, drained and chopped

- 1 red onion, chopped

- 4 garlic cloves, minced

- ½ cup apricots, cut into quarters

- 15 ounces canned chickpeas, drained

- 1 tablespoon cilantro, chopped

DIRECTIONS

In your slow cooker, combine the meat with the stock, ginger, and the rest of the ingredients except the cilantro and the chickpeas, put the lid on, and cook on Low for 7 hours and 40 minutes.

Add the cilantro and the chickpeas, cook the stew on low for 20 minutes more, divide into bowls and serve.

NUTRITION: Calories 283, Fat 11.9g, Fiber 4.5g, Carbs 28.8g, Protein 25.4g

Yogurt Marinated Pork Chops

Servings: 6

Preparation time: 2 Hours

INGREDIENTS

6 pork chops

1 cup plain yogurt

1 mandarin, sliced

2 garlic cloves, chopped

1 red pepper, chopped

Salt and pepper to taste

DIRECTIONS

1. Season the pork with salt and pepper and mix it with the remaining ingredients in a zip lock bag.

2. Marinate for 1 ½ hours in the fridge.

3. Heat a grill pan over medium flame and cook the pork chops on each side until browned.

4. Serve the pork chops fresh and warm.

NUTRITION: Calories 293, Fat 20.4g, Protein 20.6g, Carbs 4.4g

Beef And Grape Sauce

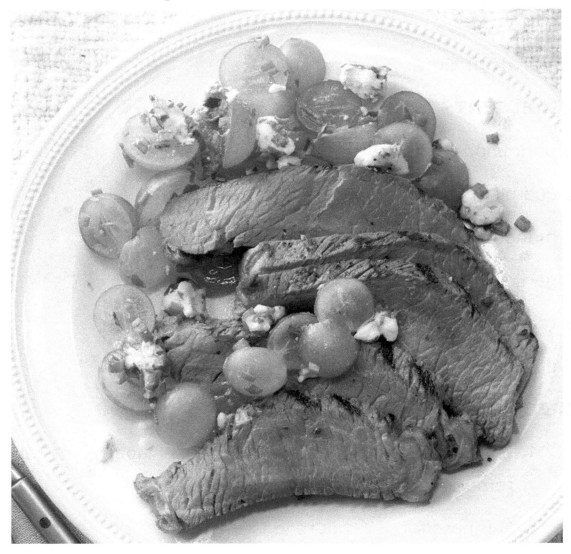

Servings: 4

Preparation time: 25 minutes

INGREDIENTS

- 1-pound beef sirloin

- 1 teaspoon molasses

- 1 tablespoon lemon zest, grated

- 1 teaspoon soy sauce

- 1 chili pepper, chopped

- ¼ teaspoon fresh ginger, minced

- 1 cup grape juice

- ½ teaspoon salt

- 1 tablespoon butter

DIRECTIONS

1. Sprinkle the beef sirloin with salt and minced ginger.

2. Heat up butter in the saucepan and add meat.

3. Roast it for 5 minutes from each side over medium heat.

4. After this, add soy sauce, chili pepper, and grape juice.

5. Then add lemon zest and simmer the meat for 10 minutes.

6. Add molasses and mix up meat well.

7. Close the lid and cook meat for 5 minutes.

8. Serve the cooked beef with grape juice sauce.

NUTRITION: Calories 267, Fat 10g, Fiber 0.2g, Carbs 7.4g, Protein 34.9g

Lamb And Tomato Sauce

Servings: 3

Preparation time: 55 minutes

INGREDIENTS

- 9 oz lamb shanks
- 1 onion, diced
- 1 carrot, diced
- 1 tablespoon olive oil
- 1 teaspoon salt
- 1 teaspoon ground black pepper
- 1 ½ cup chicken stock
- 1 tablespoon tomato paste

DIRECTIONS

Sprinkle the lamb shanks with salt and ground black pepper.

Heat up olive oil in the saucepan.

Add lamb shanks and roast them for 5 minutes from each side.

Transfer meat to the plate.

After this, add onion and carrot to the saucepan.

Roast the vegetables for 3 minutes.

Add tomato paste and mix up well.

Then add chicken stock and bring the liquid to a boil.

Add lamb shanks, stir well and close the lid.

Cook the meat for 40 minutes over medium-low heat.

NUTRITION: Calories 232, Fat 11.3g, Fiber 1.7g, Carbs 7g, Protein 25g

Lamb And Sweet Onion Sauce

Servings: 4

Preparation time: 40 minutes

INGREDIENTS

- 2 pounds lamb meat, cubed
- 1 tablespoon sweet paprika
- Salt and black pepper to the taste
- 1 and ½ cups veggie stock
- 4 garlic cloves, minced
- 2 tablespoons olive oil
- 1 pound sweet onion, chopped
- 1 cup balsamic vinegar

DIRECTIONS

1. Heat up a pot with the oil over medium heat, add the onion, vinegar. salt and pepper, stir, and cook for 10 minutes.

2. Add the meat and the rest of the ingredients. Toss, bring to a simmer, and cook over medium heat for 30 minutes.

3. Divide the mix between plates and serve.

NUTRITION: Calories 303, Fat 12.3g, Fiber 7g, Carbs 15g, Protein 17g

Pork And Mustard Shallots Mix

Servings: 4

Preparation time: 25 minutes

INGREDIENTS

3 shallots, chopped

1 pound pork loin, cut into strips

½ cup veggie stock

2 tablespoons olive oil

A pinch of salt and black pepper

2 teaspoons mustard

1 tablespoon parsley, chopped

DIRECTIONS

Heat up a pan with the oil over medium-high heat, add the shallots and sauté for 5 minutes.

Add the meat and cook for 10 minutes tossing it often.

Add the rest of the ingredients, toss, cook for 10 minutes more, divide between plates and serve right away.

NUTRITION: Calories 296, Fat 12.5g, Fiber 9.3g, Carbs 13.3g, Protein 22.5g

Basil And Shrimp Quinoa

Servings: 1 Cup

Preparation time: 20 minutes

INGREDIENTS

3 TB. extra-virgin olive oil

2 TB. minced garlic

1 cup fresh broccoli florets

3 stalk asparagus, chopped

4 cups chicken or vegetable broth

½ tsp. salt

1 tsp. ground black pepper

1 TB. lemon zest

2 cups red quinoa

½ cup fresh basil, chopped

DIRECTIONS:

1. ½ lb. medium raw shrimp (18 to 20), shells and veins removed

2. In a 2-quart pot over low heat, heat extra-virgin olive oil. Add garlic and cook for 3 minutes.

3. Increase heat to medium, add broccoli and asparagus, and cook for 2 minutes.

4. Add chicken broth, salt, black pepper, lemon zest, and bring to a boil. Stir in red quinoa, cover, and cook for 15 minutes.

5. Fold in basil and shrimp, cover, and cook for 10 minutes.

6. Remove from heat, fluff with a fork, cover, and set aside for 10 minutes. Serve warm.

NUTRITION Calories 128, Fat 12g, Fiber 6g, Protein 29g, Carbs 18g

Ground Pork Salad

Servings: 8

Preparation time: 15 minutes

INGREDIENTS

- 1 cup ground pork
- ½ onion, diced
- 4 bacon slices
- 1 teaspoon sesame oil
- 1 teaspoon butter
- 1 cup lettuce, chopped
- 1 tablespoon lemon juice
- 4 eggs, boiled
- ½ teaspoon salt
- 1 teaspoon chili pepper
- ¼ teaspoon liquid honey

DIRECTIONS

1. Make burgers: in the mixing bowl, combine together ground pork, diced onion, salt, and chili pepper.

2. Blake the medium size burgers.

3. Melt butter in the skillet and add prepared burgers.

4. Roast them for 5 minutes from each side over medium heat.

5. When the burgers are cooked, chill them a little.

6. Place the bacon in the skillet and roast it until golden brown. Then chill the bacon and chop it roughly.

7. In the salad bowl, combine together chopped bacon, sesame oil, lettuce, lemon juice, and honey. Mix up salad well.

8. Peel the eggs and cut them on the halves.

9. Arrange the eggs and burgers over the salad. Don't mix salad anymore.

NUTRITION: Calories 213, Fat 15.5g, Fiber 0.1g, Carbs 1.5g, Protein 16.5g

Beef And Dill Mushrooms

Servings: 3

Preparation time: 35 minutes

INGREDIENTS

1 cup cremini mushrooms, sliced

4 oz beef loin, sliced onto the wedges

1 tablespoon olive oil

1 teaspoon dried oregano

½ cup of water

¼ cup cream

1 teaspoon tomato paste

1 teaspoon ground black pepper

1 teaspoon salt

1 tablespoon fresh dill, chopped

DIRECTIONS

In the saucepan, combine together olive oil and cremini mushrooms.

Add dried oregano, ground black pepper, salt and dill. Mix up.

Cook the mushrooms for 2-3 minutes and add sliced beef loin.

Cook the ingredients for 5 minutes over medium heat.

After this, add cream, water, tomato paste, and mix up the meal

Simmer the beef stroganoff for 25 minutes over the medium heat

NUTRITION: Calories 196, Fat 11.8g, Fiber 0.8g, Carbs 3.5g, Protein 20g

Beef Pitas

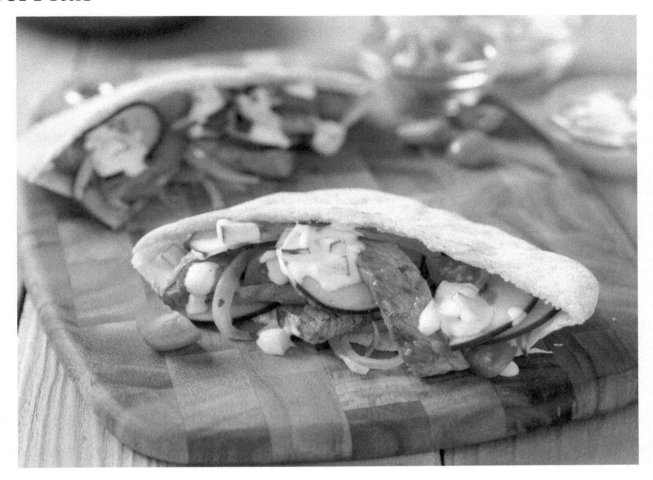

Servings: 4

Preparation time: 15 minutes

INGREDIENTS

- 1 ½ cup ground beef

- ½ red onion, diced

- 1 teaspoon minced garlic

- ¼ cup fresh spinach, chopped

- 1 teaspoon salt

- ½ teaspoon chili pepper

- 1 teaspoon dried oregano

- 1 teaspoon fresh mint, chopped

- 4 tablespoons Plain yogurt

- 1 cucumber, grated

- ½ teaspoon dill

- ½ teaspoon garlic powder

- 4 pitta bread

DIRECTIONS

1. In the mixing bowl, combine together ground beef, onion, minced garlic, spinach, salt, chili pepper, and dried oregano.

2. Blake the medium size balls from the meat mixture.

3. Line the baking tray with baking paper and arrange the meatballs inside.

4. Bake the meatballs for 15 minutes at 375F. Flip them on another side after 10 minutes of cooking.

5. Meanwhile, make tzatziki: combine together fresh mint, yogurt, grated cucumber, dill, and garlic powder. Whisk the mixture for 1 minute.

6. When the meatballs are cooked, place the over pitta bread and top with tzatziki.

NUTRITION: Calorie 253, Fat 7g, Fiber 4g, Carbs 30g, Protein 16.3g

Rosemary Lamb

Servings: 4

Preparation time: 6 Hours

INGREDIENTS

- 2 pounds lamb shoulder, cubed
- 1 tablespoon rosemary, chopped
- 3 garlic cloves, minced
- ½ cup lamb stock
- 4 bay leaves
- Salt and black pepper to the taste

DIRECTIONS

1. In your slow cooker. combine the lamb with the rosemary and the rest of the ingredients. put the lid on and cook on High for 6 hours.

2. Divide the mix between palates and serve.

NUTRITION: Info: Calories 290, Fat 13g, Fiber 11.6g, Carbs 18.3g, Protein 14g

Rosemary Creamy Beef

Servings: 4

Preparation time: 50 minutes

INGREDIENTS

2 lbs beef stem meat. cubed

2 tbsp fresh parsley, chopped

1 tsp garlic, minced

½ tsp dried rosemary

1 tsp chili powder

1 cup beef stock

1 cup heavy cream

1 onion, chopped

1 tbsp olive oil Pepper

Salt

DIRECTIONS

1. Add oil into the instant pot and set the pot on sauté mode.

2. Add rosemary, garlic, onion, and chili powder and sauté for 5 minutes.

3. Add meat and cook for 5 minutes.

4. Add remaining ingredients and stir well.

5. Seal pot with lid and cook on high for 30 minutes.

6. Once done, allow to release pressure naturally for 10 minutes, then release remaining using quick release. Remo e lid.

7. Serve and enjoy.

NUTRITION: Calories 575, Fat 29g, Carbs 4.3g, Sugar 1.3g, Protein 70.6g, Cholesterol 244mg

Mouth-Watering Lamb Stew

Servings: 4

Preparation time: 180 minutes

INGREDIENTS

- ½ cup golden raisins

- 1 cup dates, cut in half

- 1 cup dried figs, cut in half

- 1 lb lamb shoulder, trimmed of fat and cut into 2-inch cubes

- 1 onion, minced

- 1 tbsp fresh coriander

- 1 tbsp honey, optional

- 1 tbsp olive oil

- 1 tbsp Ras el Hanout

- 2 cloves garlic, minced

- 2 cups beef stock or lamb stock

- Pepper and salt to taste

- ¼ tsp ground closes

- ½ tsp ground black pepper

- 1 tsp ground turmeric

- 1 tsp ground nutmeg

- 1 tsp ground allspice

- 1 tsp ground cinnamon

- 2 tsp ground mace

- 2 tsp ground cardamom

- 2 tsp ground ginger

- ½ tsp anise seeds

- ½ tsp ground cayenne pepper

DIRECTIONS

1. Preheat oven to 300F.

2. In a small bowl, add all Ras el Hanout ingredients and mix thoroughly. Just get what the ingredients need and store remaining in a tightly lidded spice jar.

3. On high fire, place a heavy-bottomed medium pot and heat olive oil. Once hot, brown lamb pieces on each side for around 3 to 4 minutes.

4. Lower fire to medium-high and add remaining ingredients, except for the coriander.

5. Mix well. Season with pepper and salt to taste. Cover pot and bring to a boil.

6. Once boiling, turn off the fire and pop the pot into the oven.

7. Bake uncovered for 2 to 2.5 hours or until meat is fork-tender.

8. Once the meat is tender, remove it from the oven.

9. To serve, sprinkle fresh coriander and enjoy.

NUTRITION: Calories 633, Fat 21g, Carbs 78g, Protein 33g

Beef With Tomatoes

Servings: 4

Preparation time: 40 minutes

INGREDIENTS

2 lb beef roast, sliced

1 tbsp chives, chopped

1 tsp garlic, minced

½ tsp chili powder

2 tbsp olive oil

1 onion, chopped

1 cup beef stock

1 tbsp oregano, chopped

1 cup tomatoes, chopped

Pepper

Salt

DIRECTIONS

1. Add oil into the instant pot and set the pot on sauté mode.

2. Add garlic, onion, and chili powder and sauté for 5 minutes.

3. Add meat and cook for 5 minutes.

4. Add remaining ingredients and stir well.

5. Seal pot with lid and cook on high for 30 minutes.

6. Once done, allow to release pressure naturally for 10 minutes, then release remaining using quick release. Remove lid.

7. Stir well and serve.

NUTRITION: Calories 510, Fat 21.6, Carbs 5.6g, Sugar 2.5g, Protein 70g, Cholesterol 203mg

Lamb And Peanuts Mix

Servings: 4

Preparation time: 20 minutes

INGREDIENTS

- 2 tablespoons lime juice

- 1 tablespoon balsamic vinegar

- 5 garlic cloves, minced

- 2 tablespoons olive oil

- Salt and black pepper to the taste

- 1 and ½ pound lamb meat, cubed

- 3 tablespoons peanuts, toasted and chopped

- 2 scallions, chopped

DIRECTIONS

1. Heat up a pan with the oil over medium-high heat, add the meat, and cook for 4 minutes on each side.

2. Add the scallions and the garlic and sauté for 2 minutes more.

3. Add the rest of the ingredients, toss, cook for 10 minutes more, divide between plates, and serve right away.

NUTRITION: Calories 300, Fat 14.5g, Fiber 9g, Carbs 15.7g, Protein 17.5g

Cheddar Lamb And Zucchinis

Servings: 4

Preparation time: 30 minutes

INGREDIENTS

1 pound lamb meat, cubed

1 tablespoon avocado oil

2 cups zucchinis, chopped

½ cup red onion, chopped

Salt and black pepper to the taste

15 ounces canned roasted tomatoes, crushed

¾ cup cheddar cheese, shredded

DIRECTIONS

1. Heat up a pan with the oil over medium-high heat, add the meat and the onion, and brown for 5 minutes.

2. Add the rest of the ingredients except the cheese, bring to a simmer and cook over medium heat for 20 minutes.

3. Add the cheese, cook everything for 3 minutes more, divide between plates and serve.

NUTRITION: Calories 306, Fat 16.4g, Fiber 12.3g, Carbs 15.5g, Protein 18.5g

Fennel Pork

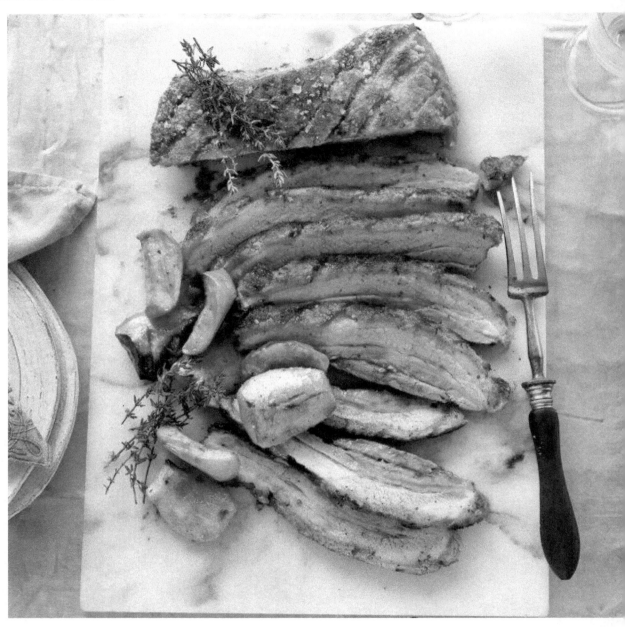

Servings: 4

Preparation time: 2 Hours

INGREDIENTS

- 2 pork loin roast, trimmed and boneless

- Salt and black pepper to the taste

- 3 garlic cloves. minced

- 2 teaspoons fennel, around

- 1 tablespoon fennel seeds

- 2 teaspoons red pepper, crushed

- ¼ cup olive oil

DIRECTIONS

1. In a roasting pan, combine the pork with salt, pepper, and the rest of the ingredients, toss, introduce in the oven and bake at 38 degrees F for 2 hours.

2. Slice the roast, divide between plates and serve with a side salad.

NUTRITION: Calories 300, Fat 4g, Fiber 2g, Carbs 6g, Protein 15g

Lamb And Feta Artichokes

Servings: 6

Preparation time: 8 Hours

INGREDIENTS

- 2 pounds lamb shoulder
- 2 spring onions, chopped
- 1 tablespoon olive oil
- 3 Garlic cloves, minced
- 1 tablespoon lemon juice
- Salt and black pepper to the taste
- 1 and ½ cups veggie stock
- 6 ounces canned artichoke hearts. drained and quartered
- ½ cup feta cheese, crumbled
- 2 tablespoons parsley, chopped

DIRECTIONS

1. Heat up a pan with the oil over medium-high heat, add the lamb, brown for 5 minutes, and transfer to your slow cooker.

2. Add the rest of the ingredients except the parsley and the cheese, put the lid on, and cook on low for 8 hours.

3. Add the cheese and the parsley, divide the mix between plates and serve.

NUTRITION: Calories 330, Fat 14.5g, Fiber 14.1g, Carbs 21.7g, Protein 17.5g

Lamb And Plums Mix

Servings: 4

Preparation time: 6 Hours and 10 minutes

INGREDIENTS

- 4 lamb shanks
- 1 red onion, chopped
- 2 tablespoons olive oil
- 1 cup plums, pitted and halved
- 1 tablespoon sweet paprika
- 2 cups chicken stock
- Salt and pepper to the taste

DIRECTIONS

1. Heat up a pan with the oil over medium-high heat, add the lamb, brown for 5 minutes on each side, and transfer to your slot cooker.

2. Add the rest of the ingredients, put the lid on, and cook on High for 6 hours.

3. Divide the mix between plates and serve right away.

NUTRITION: Calories 295, Fat 13g, Fiber 9.7g, Carbs 15.7g, Protein 14.3g

Lamb And Mango Sauce

Servings: 4

Preparation time: 1 Hour

INGREDIENTS

2 cups Greek yogurt

1 cup mango, peeled and cubed

1 yellow onion, chopped

1/3 cup parsley, chopped

1 pound lamb, cubed

½ teaspoon red pepper Blakes

Salt and black pepper to the taste

2 tablespoons olive oil

¼ teaspoon cinnamon powder

DIRECTIONS

1. Heat up a pan with the oil over medium-high heat, add the meat, and brown for 5 minutes.

2. Add the onion and sauté for 5 minutes more.

3. Add the rest of the ingredients, toss, bring to a simmer and cook over medium heat for 45 minutes.

4. Divide everything between plates and serve.

NUTRITION: Calories 300, Fat 15.3g, Fiber 9.1g, Carbs 15.8g, Protein 15.5g

Pork Chops And Cherries Mix

Servings: 4

Preparation time: 12 minutes

INGREDIENTS

4 pork chops. boneless

Salt and black pepper to the taste

½ cup cranberry juice

1 and ½ teaspoons spin mustard

½ cup dark cherries, pitted and halved

Cooling spray

DIRECTIONS

1. Heat up a pan greased with the cooking spray over medium-high heat, add the pork chops, cook them for 5 minutes on each side, and divide between plates.

2. Heat up the same pan over medium heat, add the cranberry juice and the rest of the ingredients, whisk, bring to a simmer, cook for 2 minutes, drizzle over the pork chops and serve.

NUTRITION: Calories 262g, Fat 8g, Fiber 1g, Carbs 16g, Protein 30g

Lambo And Barley Mix

Servings: 4

Preparation time: 8 Hours

INGREDIENTS

- 2 tablespoons olive oil
- 1 cup barley soaked overnight, drained, and rinsed
- 1 pound lamb meat, cubed
- 1 red onion, chopped
- 4 garlic cloves, minced
- 3 carrots, chopped
- 6 tablespoons dill, chopped
- 2 tablespoons tomato paste
- 3 cups veggie stock
- A pinch of salt and black pepper

DIRECTIONS

1. Heat up a pan with the oil over medium-high heat, add the meat, brown for 5 minutes on each side and transfer to your slot cooker

2. Add the barley, the rest of the ingredients and put the lid on, and cook on low for 8 hours.

3. Divide everything between plates and serve.

NUTRITION: Calories 292g, Fat 12g, Fiber 8.7g, Carbs 16.7, Protein 7.2g

Cashew Beef Stir Fry

Servings: 8

Preparation time: 15 minutes

INGREDIENTS

- ¼ cup coconut aminos
- 1 ½ pound ground beef
- 1 cup raw cashews
- 1 green bell pepper, julienned
- 1 red bell pepper, julienned
- 1 small can water chestnut, sliced
- 1 onion, sliced
- 1 tablespoon garlic, minced
- 2 tablespoon ginger, grated
- 2 teaspoon coconut oil
- Salt and pepper to taste

DIRECTIONS

1. Heat a skillet over medium heat, then add raw cashews. Toast for a couple of minutes or until slightly brown. Set aside.

2. In the same skillet, add the coconut oil and sauté the ground beef for 5 minutes or until brow.

3. Add the garlic, ginger and season with coconut aminos. Stir for one minute before adding the onions, bell peppers, and water chestnuts. Cook until the vegetables are almost soft.

4. Season with salt and pepper to taste.

5. Add the toasted cashews last.

NUTRITION: Calories 325, Fat 22g, Carbs 12.4g, Protein 19g

Lamb And Zucchini Mix

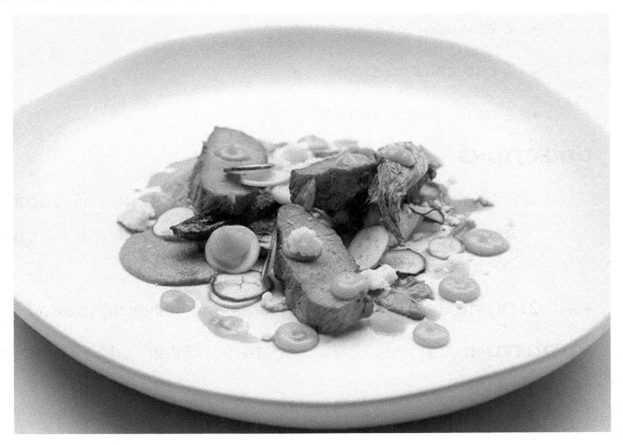

Servings: 4

Preparation Time: 4 Hours

INGREDIENTS

- 2 pounds lamb stew meat, cubed

- 1 and ½ tablespoons avocado oil

- 3 zucchinis, sliced

- 1 brown onion, chopped

- 3 garlic cloves, minced

- 1 tablespoon thyme, dried

- 2 teaspoons sage, dried

- 1 cup chicken stock

- 2 tablespoons tomato paste

DIRECTIONS

1. In a slow cooker, combine the lamb with the oil, zucchinis, and the rest of the ingredients, toss, put the lid on and cook on High for 4 hours.

2. Divide the mix between plates and serve right away.

NUTRITION: Calories 270, Fat 14.5g, Fiber 10g, Carbs 20g, Protein 13.3g

Pork And Green Beans Mix

Servings: 3

Preparation time: 35 minutes

INGREDIENTS

1 cup ground pork

1 sweet pepper, chopped

1 oz green beans, chopped

½ onion, sliced

2 oz Parmesan, grated

¼ cup chicken stock

1 teaspoon olive oil

½ teaspoon cayenne pepper

1 teaspoon dried oregano

½ teaspoon dried basil

1 teaspoon paprika

½ cup crushed tomatoes, canned

DIRECTIONS

1. Pour olive oil into the saucepan and heat it up.

2. Add ground pork and cook it for 2 minutes.

3. Then stir it carefully and sprinkle with cayenne pepper, dried oregano, dried basil, and paprika.

4. Roast the meat for 5 minutes more and add green beans, sweet pepper, and sliced onion.

5. Add chicken stock and crushed tomatoes.

6. Mix up the ground pork and close the lid.

7. Cook the meal for 20 minutes over medium heat. Stir it from time to time.

8. Then sprinkle the bolognese meat with Parmesan and mix up well.

9. Cook the meal for 5 minutes more.

NUTRITION: Calories 257, Fat 16.6g, Fiber 1.9g, Carbs 6.2g, Protein 20.9g

Artichoke Beef Roast

Servings: 6

Preparation time: 45 minutes

INGREDIENTS

- 2 lbs beef roast, cubed
- 1 tbsp garlic, minced
- 1 onion, chopped
- ½ tsp paprika
- 1 tbsp parsley, chopped
- 2 tomatoes, chopped
- 1 tbsp capers, chopped
- 10 oz can artichokes, drained and chopped
- 2 cups chicken stock
- 1 tbsp olive oil
- Pepper
- Salt

DIRECTIONS

1. Add oil into the instant pot and set the pot on sauté mode.

2. Add garlic and onion and sauté for 5 minutes.

3. Add meat and cook until brown.

4. Add remaining ingredients and stir well.

5. Seal pot with lid and cook on high for 35 minutes.

6. Once done, allow to release pressure naturally. Remove lid. Serve and enjoy.

NUTRITION: Calories 345, Fat 12g, Carbs 9.2g, Sugar 2.6g, Protein 49g, Cholesterol 135mg

Thyme Beef Round Roast

Servings: 8

Preparation time: 1 hour

INGREDIENTS

- 4 lbs beef bottom round roast, cut into pieces
- 2 tbsp honey
- 5 fresh thyme sprigs
- 2 cups red wine
- 1 lb carrots, cut into chunks
- 2 cups chicken broth
- 6 garlic cloves, smashed
- 1 onion, diced
- ¼ cup olive oil
- 2 lbs potatoes, peeled and cut into chunks
- Pepper
- Salt

DIRECTIONS

1. Add all ingredients except carrots and potatoes into the instant pot.

2. Seal pot with lid and cook on high for 45 minutes.

3. Once done., release pressure using quick release. Remove lid.

4. Add carrots and potatoes and stir well.

5. Seal pot again with lid and cook on high for 10 minutes.

6. Once done, allow to release pressure naturally. Remove lid.

7. Stir well and serve.

NUTRITION: Calories 648, Fat 21.7g, Carbs 33g, Sugar 9.7g, Protein 67g, Cholesterol 200mg

Oregano And Pesto Lamb

Servings: 4

Preparation time: 25 minutes

INGREDIENTS

- 2 pounds pork shoulder, boneless and cubed
- ¼ cup olive oil
- 2 teaspoons oregano, dried
- ¼ cup lemon juice
- 3 garlic cloves, minced
- 2 teaspoons basil pesto
- Salt and black pepper to the taste

DIRECTIONS

1. Heat up a pan with the oil over medium-high heat, add the pork, and brown for 5 minutes.
2. Add the rest of the ingredients, cook for 20 minutes more, tossing the mix from time to time, divide between plates and serve.

NUTRITION: Calories 297, Fat 14.5g, Fiber 9.3g, Carbs 16.8g, Protein 22.2g

Italian Beef Roast

Servings: 6

Preparation time: 50 minutes

INGREDIENTS

- 2 ½ lbs beef roast, cut into chunks
- 1 cup chicken broth
- 1 cup red mine
- 2 tbsp Italian seasoning
- 2 tbsp olive oil
- 1 bell pepper, chopped
- 2 celery stalks, chopped
- 1 tsp garlic, minced
- 1 onion, sliced
- Pepper
- Salt

DIRECTIONS

1. Add oil into the instant pot and set the pot on sauté mode.
2. Add the meat into the pot and sauté until brown.
3. Add onion, bell pepper, and celery and sauté for 5 minutes.

4. Add remaining ingredients and stir well.

5. Seal pot with lid and cook on high for 40 minutes.

6. Once done, allow to release pressure naturally. Remove lid. Stir well and serve.

NUTRITION: Calories 460, Fat 18.2g, Carbs 5.3g, Sugar 2.7g, Protein 58.7g, Chol 172mg

Chili Pork Meatballs

Servings: 4

Preparation time: 20 minutes

INGREDIENTS

1 pound pork meat, ground

½ cup parsley, chopped

1 cup yellow onion, chopped

4 garlic cloves, minced

1 tablespoon ginger, grated

1 Thai chili, chopped

2 tablespoons olive oil

1 cup veggie stock

2 tablespoons sweet paprika

DIRECTIONS

1. In a bowl, mix the pork with the other ingredients except for the oil, stock and paprika, stir well and shape medium meatballs out of this mix.

2. Heat up a pan with the oil over medium-high heat, add the meatballs and cook for 4 minutes on each side.

3. Add the stock and the paprika, toss gently, simmer everything over medium heat for 12 minutes more. Divide into bowls and serve.

NUTRITION: Calories 224, Fat 18g, Fiber 9.3g, Carbs 11.3g, Protein 14.4g

Square Meat Pies (Sfeeha)

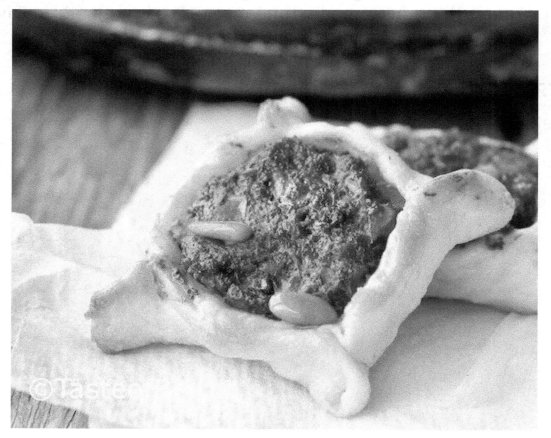

Servings: 1

Preparation time: 20 minutes

INGREDIENTS

- 1 large yellow onion

- 2 large tomatoes

- 1 lb. ground beef

- ¼ tsp. ground black pepper

- ¼ tsp salt

- 1 tsp. seven spices

- 1 batch Multipurpose Dough

DIRECTIONS

1. Preheat the oven to 425F.

2. In a food processor fitted with a chopping blade, pulse yellow onion, and tomatoes for 30 seconds.

3. Transfer tomato-onion mixture to a large bowl. Add beef, salt, black pepper, and seven spices and mix well.

4. Form Multipurpose Dough into 18 balls and roll out to 4-inch circles. Spoon 2 tablespoons of meat mixture onto the center of each dough circle. Pinch together the two opposite sides of dough up to meat mixture and pinch the opposite two sides together, forming a square. Place meat pies on a baking sheet and bake for 20 minutes.

5. Serve warm or at room temperature.

NUTRITION Calories 497, Fat 26g, Protein 34g, Carbs 38g, Fiber 9g

Lamb And Wine Sauce

Servings: 6

Preparation time: 2 Hours and 40 minutes

INGREDIENTS

- 2 tablespoons olive oil
- 2 pounds leg of lamb, trimmed and sliced
- 3 garlic cloves, chopped
- 2 yellow onions, chopped
- 3 cups veggie stock
- 2 cups dry red wine
- 2 tablespoons tomato paste
- 4 tablespoons avocado oil
- 1 teaspoon thyme, chopped
- Salt and black pepper to the taste

DIRECTIONS

1. Heat up a pan with the oil over medium-high heat, add the meat, brown for 5 minutes on each side, and transfer to a roasting pan.

2. Heat up the pan again over medium heat, add the avocado oil, add the onions and garlic and sauté for 5 minutes.

3. Add the remaining ingredients, stir, bring to a simmer and cook for 10 minutes.

4. Pour the sauce over the meat, introduce the pan in the oven, and bake at 370 degrees F for 2 hours and 20 minutes.

5. Divide onto plates and serve.

NUTRITION: Calories 273, Fat 21g, Fiber 11.1g, Carbs 16.2g, Protein 18g

Pork Meatloaf

Servings: 6

Preparation time: 1 Hour and 20 minutes

INGREDIENTS

1 red onion, chopped

Cooling spray

2 garlic cloves, minced

2 pounds pork stem, ground

1 cup almond milk

¼ cup feta cheese, crumbled

2 eggs, whisked

1/3 cup kalamata olives, pitted and chopped

4 tablespoons oregano, chopped

Salt and black pepper to the taste

DIRECTIONS

1. In a bowl, mix the meat with the onion, garlic, and the other ingredients except for the cooking spray, stir well, shape sour meatloaf, and put it in a loaf pan greased with a cooking spray.

2. Bake the meatloaf at 370 degrees F for 1 hour and 20 minutes.

3. Serve the meatloaf warm.

NUTRITION: Calories 350, Fat 23g, Fiber 1g, Carbs 17g, Protein 24g

Lamb And Rice

Servings: 4

Preparation time: 1 Hour and 10 minutes

INGREDIENTS

1 tablespoon lime juice

1 yellow onion, chopped

1 pound lamb, cubed

1 ounce avocado oil

2 garlic cloves, minced

Salt and black pepper to the taste

2 cups veggie stock

1 cup brown rice

A handful of parsley, chopped

DIRECTIONS

Heat up a pan with the avocado oil over medium-high heat, add the onion, stir and sauté for 5 minutes.

Add the meat and brown for 5 minutes more.

Add the rest of the ingredients except the parsley, bring to a simmer and cook over medium heat for 1 hour.

Add the parsley, toss, divide everything between plates, and serve.

NUTRITION: Calories 302, Fat 13g, Fiber 10.7g, Carbs 15.7g, Protein 14.3g

Italian Beef

Servings: 4

Preparation time: 35 minutes

INGREDIENTS

- 1 lb ground beef
- 1 tbsp olive oil
- ½ cup mozzarella cheese, shredded
- ½ cup tomato puree
- 1 tsp basil
- 1 tsp oregano
- ½ onion, chopped
- 1 carrot, chopped
- 14 oz can tomatoes, diced
- Pepper
- Salt

DIRECTIONS

Add oil into the instant pot and set the pot on sauté mode.

Add onion and sauté for 2 minutes.

Add meat and sauté until bronzed.

Add remaining ingredients except for cheese and stir well.

Seal pot with lid and cook on high for 35 minutes.

Once done, release pressure using quick release. Remove lid.

Add cheese and stir well and cook on sauté mode until cheese is melted.

Serve and enjoy.

NUTRITION: Calorie 298, Fat 11.3g, Carbs 11g, Sugar 6.2g, Protein 37g, Chol 103mg

Pork Chops And Peppercorns Mix

Servings: 4

Preparation time: 20 minutes

INGREDIENTS

1 cup red onion, sliced

1 tablespoon black peppercorns, crushed

¼ cup veggie stock

5 garlic cloves, minced

A pinch of salt and black pepper

2 tablespoons olive oil

4 pork chops

DIRECTIONS

1. Heat up a pan with the oil over medium-high heat, add the pork chops, and brown for 4 minutes on each side.

2. Add the onion and the garlic and cook for 2 minutes more.

3. Add the rest of the ingredients, cook everything for 10 minutes, tossing the mix from time to time, divide between plates and serve.

NUTRITION: Calories 232, Fat 9.2g, Fiber 5.6g, Carbs 13.3g, Protein 24.2g

Pork And Tomato Meatloaf

Servings: 8

Preparation time: 55 minutes

INGREDIENTS

- 2 cups ground pork
- 1 egg, beaten
- ¼ cup crushed tomatoes
- 1 teaspoon salt
- 1 teaspoon ground black pepper
- 1 oz Swiss cheese, grated
- 1 teaspoon minced garlic
- 1/3 onion, diced
- ¼ cup black olives, chopped
- 1 jalapeno pepper, chopped
- 1 teaspoon dried basil
- Cooking spray

DIRECTIONS

Spray the loaf mold with cooking spray.

Then combine together ground pork, egg, crushed tomatoes, salt, ground black pepper. Grated Swiss cheese, minced garlic, onion, olives, jalapeno pepper and dried basil.

Stir the mass until it is homogenous and transfer it to the prepared load mold.

Flatten the surface of the meatloaf well and cover with foil.

Bake the meatloaf for 40 minutes at 375F.

Then discard the foil and bake the meal for 15 minutes more.

Chill the cooked meatloaf to room temperature and then remove it from the loaf mold.

Slice it on the servings.

NUTRITION: Calories 263, Fat 18.3g, Fiber 0.6g, Carbs 1.9g, Protein 22g

Beef And Eggplant Moussaka

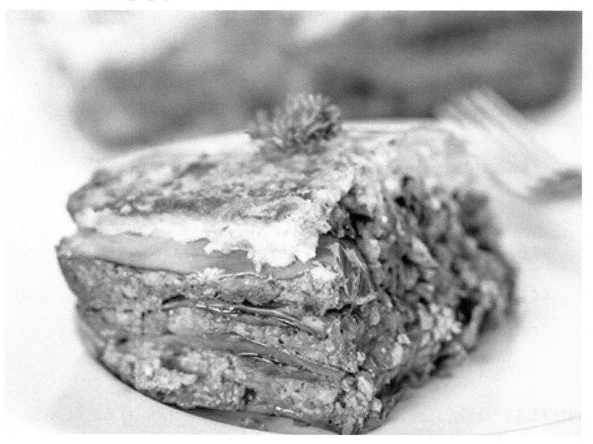

Servings: 3

Preparation time: 50 minutes

INGREDIENTS

- 1 small eggplant, sliced

- 1 teaspoon olive oil

- ½ cup cream

- 1 egg, beaten

- 1 tablespoon wheat flour, whole grain

- 1 teaspoon cornstarch

- 3 oz Romano cheese, grated

- ½ cup ground beef

- ¼ teaspoon minced garlic

- 1 tablespoon Italian parsley, chopped

- 3 tablespoons tomato sauce

- ¾ teaspoon ground nutmeg

DIRECTIONS

1. Sprinkle the eggplants with olive oil and ground nutmeg and arrange them in the casserole mold in one layer.

2. After this, place the ground beef in the skillet.

3. Add minced garlic, Italian parsley, and ground nutmeg.

4. Then add tomato sauce and mix up the mixture well.

5. Roast it for 10 minutes over medium heat.

6. Make the sauce: in the saucepan, whisk together cream with egg.

7. Bring the liquid to boil (simmer it constantly) and add wheat flour, cornstarch and cheese. Stir well.

8. Bring the liquid to boil and stir till cheese is melted. Remove the sauce from the heat.

9. Put the cooked ground beef over the eggplants and flatten well.

10. Pour the cream sauce over the ground beef.

11. Cover the meal with foil and secure the edges.

12. Bake moussaka for 30 minutes at 365F.

NUTRITION: Calories 270, Fat 16.1g, Fiber 5.9g, Carbs 15.4g, Protein 17.6g

Hearty Meat And Potatoes

Servings: 2 Cups

Preparation time: 30 minutes

INGREDIENTS

- 1 lb. ground beef or lamb

- ¼ cup extra-Virgin olive oil

- 1 large yellow onion, chopped

- 5 large potatoes, peeled and cubed

- ½ tsp salt

- 1 TB. seven spices

- ½ tsp. ground black pepper

DIRECTIONS

1. In a large, 3-quart pot over medium heat, brown beef for 5 minutes, breaking up chunks with a wooden spoon.

2. Add extra-Virgin olive oil and yellow onion, and cook for 5 minutes.

3. Toss in potatoes, salt, seven spices, and black pepper. Cover and cook for 10 minutes. Toss gently, and cook for 10 more minutes.

4. Serve warm with a side of Greek yogurt.

NUTRITION Calories 412, Fat 7g, Protein 19g, Carbs 81g, Fiber 9g

Ita Sandwiches

Servings: 1 Pita Sandwich

Preparation time: 20 minutes

INGREDIENTS

- 1 lb. ground beef
- 1 tsp. salt
- ½ tsp. ground black pepper
- 1 tsp. seven spices
- 4 (6 or 7 in.) pitas

DIRECTIONS

Preheat the oven to 400°F.

In a medium bowl, combine beef, salt, black pepper, and seven spices.

Lay out pitas on the counter, and divide beef mixture evenly among them, and spread beef to the edge of pitas.

Place pitas on a baking sheet and bake for 20 minutes.

Serve warm with Greek yogurt.

NUTRITION Calories 880, Fat 45g, Carbs 71g, Fiber 3g, Protein 47g

Lamb And Dill Apples

Servings: 4

Preparation time: 25 minutes

INGREDIENTS

- 3 green apples, cored, peeled and cubed
- Juice of 1 lemon
- 1 pound lamb stew meat, cubed
- 1 small bunch of dill, chopped
- 3 ounces heavy cream
- 2 tablespoon olive oil
- Salt and black pepper to the taste

DIRECTIONS

1. Heat up a pan with the oil over medium-high heat, add the lamb, and brown for 5 minutes.

2. Add the rest of the ingredients, bring to a simmer and cook over medium heat for 20 minutes.

3. Divide the mix between plates and serve.

NUTRITION: Calories 328, Fat 16.7g, Fiber 10.5g, Carbs 21.6g, Protein 14.7g

Conclusion

I am so interested to see what tasty recipes you have actually developed.

I make sure you have actually been active and also we have actually thrilled the tastes buds of loved ones.

Do not quit working out as well as maintain attempting these meals. They are distinct, healthy and balanced as well as healthy. Perfect for the entire family members.

I constantly suggest speaking with a nutritional expert prior to any type of dietary modifications, as well as obtaining lots of exercise.

I thanks as well as eagerly anticipate future dishes.